The Metaphor

Neil Douglas-Tubb

A Journey of Healing

Copyright

This book is a work of fiction. Any references to historical events, real people, or real places are used fictitiously. Other names, characters, places, and events are products of the author's imagination, and any resemblance to actual events, places, or persons, living or dead, is entirely coincidental.

ISBN: 9781973329022
Copyright © 2017

The Metaphor-A Journey of Healing
Douglas-Tubb, Neil (1947–)

Editing by Katie Heffring
Jacket design by Neil Douglas-Tubb
Publicist
Typesetting by Katie Heffring
Printed and Bound in Canada by Kindle/Amazon

Dedication

To those who helped when everyone else ran for cover ... I thank you ... from the bottom of my heart, I thank you.

I hope that Marty and Pat know that I kept my promise "to pass it on," because Lord knows I've tried ... thank you so much for saving my life ...

NDT 2017

There is a mythical door that EXITS this universe that my consciousness seems to be focused in.

This door does not appear at the end of some hallway or corridor of my mind, but in the great hall of my awareness. It is in the very center of that enormous place. For me it is a regular door, wooden with a large gold knocker on it.

Now the odd thing is this door is always facing me. No matter where I am in my consciousness, this closed door in the center of the great hall is facing me.

I really never noticed this before because I have been too busy working out my life and existence. It seems that I had to really slow down enough just to notice it there waiting for me.

So I will wonder aloud, I wonder if my "terrible dailyness" is a way that I use not to have to face the presence of this door and its passage to places and parts unknown.

There seems to be a complicity or a willingness on my end not to grow, not to know, not to notice, to stay stagnate and the same. This doorway now invites me to grow, and to know, but in doing so, I am afraid that I will have to give up all that I am familiar with. But I "now" know that I will not have to give up all that I know.

The key phrase here seems to be "I am afraid." So having admitted that, I can look for the proof that I can venture through this door and not be torn to shreds.

Here is the proof, this door to the greater me is within me, not outside of me, and I now know that it will lead me to a greater understanding of who I am.

I also know that I will have to leave behind those things and people that I cling to for my false sense of security that I think I so desperately need.

So, I can go through that door at any time IF; I want to make the journey, and I know that; the doorway has patience enough to wait out my fears, after all it has eternity on its side; but It will not give up its' secrets unless I give over my resistance

Table of Contents

One

It has been my belief since my earliest memory that "I am alone and my world is a dangerous place". My life seems to affirm this to me daily. I have found that I only can acquire the relief and happiness that I think I want by doing something or getting something. There are times when I feel I am so desperate, lost and alone.

I have learned that when my best efforts fail me that I have gathered habits along the way that I can depend on. These habits are creations from outside of me and they are "magical". They take their form as substances, actions or facilities, things that I use daily just to get by on. I know that I can always reach out to them and they can be relied on. It is sad but true that these "magical" chattels are my addictions, obsessions and/or compulsions.

As I still my thoughts and close my eyes, I begin to realize that I have placed the scant shadow of my faith in a place and on activities that are misbegotten.

I am beginning to admit to myself that my beliefs really are not true. The various forms of my beliefs, my addictions, obsessions and/or compulsions are devices that have only brought me pain.

I am admitting that I have no control over them, in fact I have given them all my power.

I also notice that they have no power of their own. They sit there like lifeless forms, shadows or ghosts, awaiting only the wind of my restlessness to stir my soul and scatter them.

I admit that I have been insane and I begin to wonder about what may lay before me as I begin my journey toward finding the world of my sanity.

Experience has Taught Me

That I am out of control and I know I am
not happy.
That my Beliefs have not and cannot make
me happy.
I know I must find "different" to be happy.
Where will I look?
What will I see?
And who will help me?

First Principle

Live Life to the Fullest

Imagine that your life is a Dish Rag and it is wet...

And it is your lifetime commitment to squeeze every drop of water out of this dish rag until it's dry

Every opportunity then Squeeze

Two

Over and over, I have followed my own advice on what I think I should do and how I think I should do it and each time it came up the same, I have failed.

There are times when the desperation inside of me becomes so overwhelming; I don't think I can go on another moment.

But as I quiet my mind and close my eyes I notice, for the first time in years, that there is a part of me that remembers the truth of whom I am. It speaks to me in a voice that is neither male nor female and reassures that all is not for naught.

Imagine that, from deep inside me, a Voice of sanity, reassurance, comfort and truth. This is a voice that I recall from my childhood, soft and certain, it reminds me of my Maker and It tells me I am part of all that is. One with! I am part of the plan too and I belong, no longer left out.

"No Child of God, can be less than perfect."

There is warmth and a comfort that comes over me as I sense this presence deep within me. Oh, it is hard to discern at first, but each time I acknowledge it to be alive and well within me, I feel it grow and become more pronounced and defined, and more a part of my life.

I feel the pieces of me beginning to come home from their hiding places and take their rightful place within me.

The missing parts of me are beginning to fall into place, as if some giant hand is now beginning to put me, the jig saw puzzle, back together again.

. . . Experience Has Taught Me That . . .

**I know that I have many avenues open to
me and it really is a simple decision.
A or B
Choose the new and unfamiliar, take the
risks and begin to experiment with
something that I have discovered within
me, something totally new and unfamiliar
or
Do it the old way and take one more step
towards death.
Which will I choose**

Second Principle[i]

"Trust" is about value, not about pain reduction, not about expectations ... *this can slip and slide through misunderstanding into the manifestation of all my fears* ... **"Trust" is about "what has real value" ... not necessarily what I imagine it to be.**

Three

So here I stand at a junction in my mind with my soul in hand, or so it seems. Many confusing and contradicting messages seem to be presenting themselves and I feel confused. Now through this fog of imagery there is a sense to one particular way. It is not marked by anything in particular, and actually it feels just a little scary to even consider going down that road but there is a sense of something that wafts down this way of doing things that is definitely different. If peace and good order have a smell about them, then it is here.

I look to my left and see many other opportunities I could venture out into, some very familiar, heck, I could walk through some of them with my eyes shut. In fact, I see many of the old gang beckoning too me to join them in the old ways.

I feel my heart strings tug on this one. I look down this old and familiar road and I can see pain and despair hiding in the ditches just waiting to jump out at me. I see me depending on me, and my "magic friends" to gain relief from the attacks. I now know that the relief I will feel is only temporary. As I see my old friends I have to ask myself who is my friend and who is my enemy, really? Who has the false faces on today? I notice my life is littered with the castoffs of my efforts to avoid my legitimate hurt and pain.

I want 'different'. That path way to the unfamiliar looks different. I notice others up ahead. They seem to be walking with a spring in their step, they seem to be walking toward a place called 'different'.

They are whom I want to join. We all carry heavy packsacks with us, and some of us have yokes about our necks too but I notice that their steps are light and the look upon their faces is peaceful. A sense of renewal comes upon me.

The old gang raises hell and bangs their pots and pans. They really don't want me to go. They shout promises, and falsehoods and even try bribery, offering all sorts of freedom and wonderful experiences if only I would stay. It is tempting but I don't hear the ring of quality in their voices, I remember what I have learned in the first two steps, in fact if I am honest with me I have to notice that the ring of quality it was never really there ever. I choose the road of unfamiliar and different.

Those greet me who have gone on before. The warmth and presence deep within grows deeper and richer. Gratitude becomes my experience not my lip service. I experience not being alone. I experience the presence of my Higher Power acting with me as I go through my day, as I walk upon my path.

. . . Experience Has Taught Me That . . .

There is a power great than me, and I can have it in my life but only if I ask and only if I surrender into it. Then it will heal all in my life that needs to be healed, including me.

Third Principle

Know Thy Self

Four

I seem to be pointed in an interesting direction now, but this is anything but easy, in fact it seems to be a lot like work. I seem to have a good sense of my Higher Power now but I seem to be weighed down by who and what I think I am.

Time to begin to examine who it is that I think I might be.

So, I find a place by a mystical stream and take off this metaphorical backpack and begin to examine whom it is that I think and thought I was and am.

My pack is full to overflowing with stuff. Old stuff, new stuff, embarrassing stuff, stuff I wouldn't tell anyone, even on my death bed, and stuff I don't even know that I have done. There is so much stuff, I cannot count it all. So I reach in and take hold of some stuff, a shiny sort of thing, and I begin to examine it.

I have been told to catalogue what I find, just for posterity's sake. Not too sure why, other than it sounded like something I should do and one of my fellow travelers said maybe it was a good idea. Out comes the shiny thing and I see me reflected in it and I sort of like what comes out, it shows me off to be a nice, loving sort of a person. I am actually sort of surprised, but I catalogue it and carry on.

Then out comes a handful of goop, and it is black and sticky and smelly, and I just know everyone is looking at it and I am so embarrassed by it. I catalogue it too and then set it aside.

I watch both of these items in the light of day and notice something unusual. First the goop, as it is exposed to the light of day, it dries out and slowly the smell lifts. I notice that it could be brushed off, if I wanted.

I acknowledge this, and as I do that the shiny sort of thing, the loving parts of me, begins to melt into the pores of my being and become part of what I know about myself. Interesting.

I check in with my Higher Power and I ask what should I do with all this stuff in the backpack? That Voice of Sanity tells me, with great certainty, to continue until all is examined and catalogued.

What a task; I don't think I can go through with it, but I know I have to. It is part of my ritual of surrender. It really is my first action I have had taken toward my own recovery. I carry on into my future.

. . . Experience Has Taught Me That . . .

**I am thankful for the opportunity to come
to know me**

Fourth Principle

You are responsible for you ...

Not your partner ...

Just You!

Your partner is not responsible for you.

36

Five

So here I sit next to a mystical stream or tree or something with a now empty metaphorical backpack at my side.

Now what?

I notice that there is dust covering me, and I am afraid that passersby will notice. It is embarrassing to sit here all covered in the grunge of my past. I feel shame and embarrassment. I know that everyone passing by can see and in my mind, I am sure that I know exactly what he or she is thinking. I'm afraid, and what if my newfound God might find out about me, too?

As I think those thoughts, I slowly begin to sense a feeling of warmth and certainty fill my body. I sense that I am safe again.

I can now both sense and hear that Voice, and this is a poor description of the experience, but they are the only words I can use to describe what happens when I communicate with my Higher Power.

The Voice is much a part of me now and it tells me that these things that I called "stuff" are only the things that happened to me, not who I am. Perfect, Upright and Beautiful, Somedays My Behavior Stinks I am not my Behavior. I sense or hear that this Power within me loves me for me, then I remember an old phrase, God Don't Make No Junk.

I begin to look for someone who has already walked this part of the path, someone to share with, someone who seems to know his or her way along this pathway. I know that I need to do this. I know and I want to brush off the dust. Just like cataloguing the stuff, I now know in my heart of hearts that I must unburden myself in the presence of both my Higher Power and another living breathing human being.

This feels scary but I know this must be done.

Who will I trust?

I ask for guidance from my Higher Power and as I do, I notice someone is there beside me. I look at them and just know they are the one.

Together we sift through the dust.

For the first time in my life I feel accepted and safe.

. . . Experience Has Taught Me That . . .
I Can Allow Myself To Heal
And I Am Thankful To Begin To Trust
Again
It Is The Work That I Do

Fifth Principle

Spirit and Spiritual

Six

Exhausted, I sit here pondering, what I should do next? Sitting beside me is all my mess. Do I attempt to tidy it up? Do I put things back the way they were? Will that really work any longer? What I now know is I just have to get on with getting' on down the road. As I do, I notice my step is lighter. Not totally lightened by a long shot, but lighter than it was. Better stop and meditate on what I just did. What it means to me. And what is next? I see others on the path and they don't have any baggage at all. They actually seem full of life and happy.

I begin to wish my If Only Wish; if only my burdens were gone too, then I could be just like them. As I begin my journey into self-pity. I hear the Voice again and it says to me "So you think you wish your weight should be lifted from you, do you? I respond out loud, "Yes!"

The Voice Of Certainty says, "Look at yourself, look at how you hold on to your mess; you do as if it were gold to be treasured." There I was caught in the act of being my old scared self. Hanging on for dear life to what I imagined I thought I was.

I now know, if I am to move on in my recovery, I have to let go of "My Stuff, My Hurt, My Shame and My Pain." I notice, perhaps for the first time, that I hold this mess of mine with a death grip.

The Inner Voice of Sanity tells me that no two people do this releasing thing in the same fashion. Some let go all at once and others do it a bit at a time. And some do it slowly and laboriously, sometimes stretched over entire lifetimes. And of course, some never do it. It is all up to me, to get on with my business of me finding me.

"If I can imagine," this voice tells me, "that is the first step in having something called different".

I visualize myself letting go of all the trash. The stuff I carry to identify me to me. As I take the risk to do this act of release, I feel filled with life and love.

I am relaxed. I am ready. I reflect.

Experience has Taught Me That

As I release the past in the present, in hopes of finding my future, that is the promise, I get it. Finding my future now is the only time I have to experiment with.

Sixth Principle

Be Self Soothing

Seven

So here I sit, still exhausted but clearer of mind.

I have decided deep within me that I am ready.

I have decided is the key phrase.

I am ready to let go of all this stuff, all this mess.

I close my eyes and I pray, probably for the first time in my life, I sincerely pray to my Higher Power and simply ask, "Take all this from me."

I sense the presence of that Voice again. It is here with me now, beside me and silent. I can feel it, I can't hear it, I can just feel its presence.

Then I hear.

You have no burden to remove. I did not error in your creation. You are perfect, as are all my creations. You are made in my image. I, as your maker, see only that, you are perfect in my creation, which is all there is too see for either you or me.

So, I instruct you: You made your burden; you set it down and walk away from it.

Simply leave by the side of the path. I will come in my own good time pick it up and put it to its proper use elsewhere in my creation. Simply go and leave it there for me to pick up later.

For the first time ever in my life, I know absolutely that I am not alone.

Others have stopped and they take me by my hand and we walk together toward our future.

The future Our Creator intended for us to have.

Experience Has Taught Me That

No Longer At Odds With Everything . . . I Am Free
I Am Free as God Created Me

Seventh Principle

An Exercise To Take You Into Your Future

What Beliefs Do I Follow That Lift Me Up?
What Beliefs Do I Follow That Bring Me Down?
What Beliefs Do I Follow That Are Based In Truth?
Which Of Those Beliefs Are Based On Lies?

When I notice there is something out of balance, something that brings me down, something that is a lie or out of line with the **Way of Things**, then there are only two things that are necessary.

First, make up a new rule/belief that encompasses you being uplifted. **Then Do It**.

Second, say to yourself or to whoever may be present:
I'm Sorry, Please Forgive Me. I Love You
The important thing is that you offer this up to your own soul first.

Remember:

You Act Your Way Into A New Way Of Thinking ...
Not Think Your Way Into a New Way of Acting

Eight

Well here I am walking along the path with a newfound friend. Yes, my pack is gone. I am happy, for the first time in my life I can honestly say that I am happy. No, I am not at peace with myself totally, but I am happy.

My friend tells me that I have more to do. You have to set to right those things that you set into motion that were either not centered or off balance. He told me that I had to become willing to set things straight. Wow what a task. Actually, be willing to be responsible for what I have done. Imagine that, me being responsible. I suddenly realize I had no idea what to do to be responsible. What does it mean to set things right?

Well I am told that you must become prepared and willing to deal with every person or situation about which or upon whom you have left your mark.

These may be things that you feel guilty about, or they may not, but you must be willing to deal with them in a fashion that will inspire peace to return to your relationship with them or it.

There is only one thing that I can do. I can pray and ask for guidance and begin to trust that I will get the answers that I need to hear when I need to hear them. I have begun the business of coming to terms with the fact that all persons are equal in God's eyes. My perception of this un-equalness is what fired the pit of my own pain, hurt and shame. I noticed that I had not recognized others as having a value before God.

I am beginning to understand that in the process of healing of my relationships is the healing process of my soul.

As I respect others as equal members of the Interplanetary Galactic Starship, then I am learning to respect me and all my processes. Time to write, time to journal and tell me my story and this time notice the toes I have stepped on.

Experience Has Taught Me That:

**There are others on the face of this earth
and they belong here too. I am grateful to
My Creator for providing me with the
opportunity to see this simple truth.
Imagine That, Simple Truths
Plain as day yet buried deep inside my
soul where I never looked before,**

Eighth Principle

Style
Theirs and Mine
Do we agree or are our Ego's Clashing?

Nine

Finally, things seem to be coming to completion. I've got my cataloguing done, I've made my lists and I have become willing to fix whatever it is that needs to be fixed. "I'm ready!" I shout from beside the mystical stream. "I'm ready." I'm also, very much in a hurry. Understatement! "Let's just get this thing done so I can get on with the rest of my life," I say to myself under my breath.

"Now, before anything else happens, I'll just start to get in touch with some of those lost souls I may have trudged upon and say I'm sorry. I'll knock off a few names tonight and then a few tomorrow and it will be done in nothing flat. Right!"

I feel a presence with me now. Neither male nor female, that Voice just seems to be here filling some unseen space and its other quality at this moment is that it is silent.

But I can feel it.

My newfound friend and guide asks me where I'm going. I tell him that I am off just to get a few names ticked off the list and done before nightfall, and he says "slow down. This is not what you may think it is. This is not wham bam thank you and I'm sorry ma'am. This is a process of setting things to right. So sorry does not really enter into it unless it is something that is really necessary. Remember every case is different. Sometimes you can't do anything at all."

Wise advice.

"So how will I know? And what and how to do it when I get there?" I asked.

My friend says, "Trust that your Higher Power knows what He Or She is doing. Listen for the direction you receive from Him Or Her. Remember, if you are willing to ask, then be open to listening. So many just ask and never listen."

So with a different attitude now, I take out my list, look at the first name and I pray.

Now I begin to sense that presence beside me, I sense it begin to stir. Oddly enough I seem to know what needs to be done next.

Experience Has Taught Me

Next is a worthwhile concept.

Actually, knowing what needs to be done next. I can allow the healing of my relationships if I want. I have the power within me. I am connected now. It is with me. I am part of it. Amazing.

Ninth Principle[ii]

EXPERIENCE has taught us that there are PRINCIPLES OF SHARING. I can use these principles to find out more about my world and myself.

1. Most of my partner's criticisms of me have some basis in reality. (Note the words 'some basis'; no one said 'total basis' by any stretch of the imagination.)

2. Many of my repetitive, emotional criticisms of my partner are disguised statements of my own unmet needs. Of course the same is also true for my partner. (Note the key phrase in this statement is my own unmet needs.)

3. Some of my repetitive, emotional criticisms of my partner may be an accurate description of a disowned part of me. *My Blind Spots*.

4. Some of my criticisms of my partner may help me identify my own lost self.

5. One must remember this is not about liking what you see; this is about discovering what is hidden in plain sight.

Ten

Well, I am up walking again. Heading off in the direction of the rest of my life. The sun is shining, the grass is green and the flowers smell wonderful. I'm happy with myself and I can actually say that I feel carefree, unencumbered. Now I know that I have not finished with my business of making amends, but I got a darned good start on it. It will end when it does. I know that now. I notice something else also. People enjoy being with me. Some smile at me and some twinkle a hello with their eyes. I am somebody and others actually acknowledge that as they pass by. Simply being here in the first place on a wonderful day becomes very fulfilling. I belong.

I go into a whatnot shop and browse. There is an old guy in there that looks like he has many years' practice at besting his customers.

I'm ready for old foe. My browsing pays off. There hidden at the back of the shop is an Old Group Of Seven painting being sold for the value of the frame only. $25 bucks. It is worth thousands. Imagine my good fortune. How lucky can I be all in one day! I thank God for his special gift. I purchase it and make a beeline for the door and run. Me, I'm proud of me for being so shrewd and wise and besting the old boy at his own game. Then I sense this thing beside me again. Neither Male nor Female, Just A Presence. I sense it there, very profound in its silence and I begin to recognize the truth of what I have just done. I feel ashamed. Its healthy shame.

So back to the whatnot shop I go. I fess up. I tell the old fellow what a find I made hidden at the back of his shop.

I return it for a refund. I see his eyes light up with gratitude and tears. He says to me that he has had to work all these years long past a time when most would retire because his grandson needed an education. He was the only one who could possibly provide that education. Now he can both retire and gift his grandchild what he needs to have the education he has always wanted.

For the first time in my life I am proud of my actions. Actually, I'm proud of what I have done with this old man and for myself. We shake hands in true friendship.

Experience Has Taught Me That

**When I trust my guidance, it will tell me
what to do.
Imagine that, guidance that actually works**

Tenth Principle
Hope

Hope is shared amongst us all.

It is a universal human experience which brings us together in our diversity and at the same time is a personal experience which shows differently for everyone.

Hope is a quality which is found in the stories of peoples' lives ... *not in analysis of the situation*. Our news media draws us to the tragedies and melodrama of life but we as individuals have the choice to look in another direction. It is a complex human quality which:

- **-is rooted in our past experiences;**
- **-has an orientation to the future;**
- **-is expressed in how we live today.**

Eleven

So, as I begin to move into the many tomorrows of the rest of my life I notice that I have come out of a dream-like-state, one that I had been in for most of my life. Odd, being out here in the real world. I notice that I look forward to the day ahead of me. Imagine that looking forward to what is next.

Strange thoughts for a guy like me.

So I tidy myself up just a little and turn my focus in on my Higher Power. I sort of combine prayer/conversation/meditation. I just take the time to notice and acknowledge that my God is now a part of my life and I am part of His or Her expression of the universe. So. as I acknowledge my place in God's creation, I take the time to offer and any questions about my life that I feel I need guidance on.

I toss them out into the ring and just leave them for God to deal with in His or Her own good time. It is sort of like a spiritual morning shower.

I close my eyes and turn my thoughts to my Creator.

Acknowledging the sacredness of all things, of all people. I ask simple things like: What would you have me do today? Or, let me be one of your instruments today. Place before me what you would have me do and with your strength and wisdom I will do my very best to do what needs to be done?

I notice that as I talk with my God in this fashion He actually answers me. I notice something else, that if I offer thankfulness for the as of yet immature day it becomes just a little nicer place to be no matter what happens. I no longer feel alone. I seem to get answers to questions that previously baffled me, and things actually get done that used to overwhelm me. Sometimes it's the garbage that needs to be taken out and out it goes and sometimes my job seems to be to save a soul or two, and then it is lifesaving 101. It is only what I do. I do it for and more importantly with God. I never did that before. Now it is my way of things. But it is whatever is next and it is not my agenda any longer and I can now live comfortably with me not trying to prove and re prove who it is that I thought I was.

I notice I have forgiven. Oh, it was never ok that what happened actually happened to me but that doesn't matter anymore, I've unhooked from the past and all the energy I had invested from protecting me from the ghosts of my past. I never really noticed this until now. And I am not too sure when that release happened. But it did and I am thankful for it. I now know that if I want to understand my innocence, I need to ask for the willingness to forgive.

Experience Has Taught Me Gratitude

I know for the first time that I am truly not alone

Eleventh Principle[iii]

The Way of Things

Conflict in social interaction comes in many forms: brute force, implacable institutions, and internal divisions among one's friends, fellow workers and family. If there is to be an opening in any situation, a way through to resolution, we are going to have to be willing to listen to what we have to say to ourselves about others and ourselves,

(**Ninth Principle**) and at the same time not be caught in the reactive nature that has brought us to this impasse in the first place. Don Miguel Ruiz, The Four Agreements ... **"Don't Take Things Personally."**
Insights don't come easily, as you probably are discovering. It takes a great deal of strength to detach yourself from who you think you are and be honest.

After all, we all have vested interests in whom and what we think we are and what is going on around us. What is going on around us is the stuff that gives us our definitions of who we think we are. We tend to seek out those situations, people and events that support what we have come to think about ourselves in the first place.

It's a cycle. **Nothing more, nothing less**.

Twelve

I'm well along on my path now.

I've traveled quite a piece.

I'm now doing whatever needs to be done in a fashion that it seems to need doing. And it is my belief now that as I follow my spiritual practices that all this is being done stuff is being done in conjunction with my Higher Power's will for me.

I have come to learn that I have always been in perfectly the right place for me to be, even in the face of what sometimes appears to be overwhelming evidence to the contrary, at least in my mind anyway.

It warms the cockles of my heart to have real friends, people who actually enjoy me as much I enjoy them.

My world is now a wonderful place. The grass is still green as it always was and the sun still rises in the east as it always has, but I see things so differently now.

Imagine that, knowing I am in exactly the right place at exactly the right time doing exactly the right thing. Now that is confidence isn't it.

As I come upon a mystical stream I notice someone struggling with a metaphorical backpack. I wonder what is next in line for me to day. I sit down beside him and ask, "Are you looking for someone? How Can I Help?"

Experience Has Taught Me That

**I have something very worthwhile to offer.
That is and was god plan for me all along.
I just had to go out and find it, dust it off
And
Then be prepared to just do it.**

Twelfth Principle[iv]

Your imagination is what is creating your reality.

This is True.

Curiosity motivates us to do something with what we imagine.

This is a very powerful concept.

In fact, one of the most Powerful things you own.

This Also is True.

Imagination is a force that can actually manifest reality.

Your Job is to Use It Wisely

Wisdom Comes From, Experience... Not Books ... Not Analysis

Imagine That!

Thirteenth Principle[v] (Expanded)

The respect of and for your team, your partners (Life and Business) is more important than all the laurels the world can provide.

Don't put limitations on yourself.

Don't think yourself into a place that stops you before you start.

Stay Away From "I Can't."

It doesn't work very Well.

Learn to speak your Feelings as they are.

Know this:

Being Nice is Not a Nice Thing to do, especially when you do it to you.

Others will put limitations on you.

They will drop their stuff and their opinions on you.

Don't take it personally.

And more importantly: don't do it to yourself.

Remember This:

Your best Thinking may not be your best Friend.

Don't bet against you before you start.

Learn to speak up and speak out.

Not your opinions ... your feelings.

Fourteenth Principle[vi]

Take Risks

"Failure is not an option"

This Statement Is Not True.

Failure has to be an option for life to be rich.

Why?

Simple!

It is in the **"leap of faith"** that **Risk Taking Entails**

It is here in that space of conscious awareness that life gains its flavor.

Life and its richness are embodied in the attempting to do

what you've never done before.

So failure has to be an option

But fear is not.

Fifteenth Principle
Arthur C. Clarke

The only way of discovering the limits of the
"possible" is
to venture a little way past them into the
"impossible".

About the Author

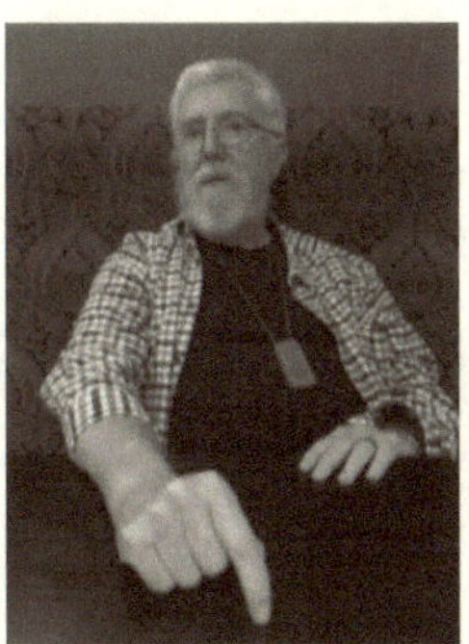

Neil is in private practice as a Registered Clinical Counselor (0396) in the Province of British Columbia, specializing in Dissociative Disorders and the treatment of Post Trauma Stress (grossing over 30,000 hours in one-on-one sessional work with clients and over 14,000 plus hours as group facilitator). He is a member of the British Columbia Association of Clinical Counselors.

In the early days before Neil was into any of this "stuff" he was a member of the Royal Canadian Mounted Police Security Service. He worked in Counter Espionage-"B"-ops—RIS, (*Russian Intelligence Service, KGB and GRU*. He stepped out of that world nearly four decades ago (*April Fools Day 1979*) and into this world to search out his own past and his own ghosts and to dust off his own future.

Michael Poole, documentary film director/maker and author, in his book *Romancing Mary Jane: A Year In The Life Of A Failed Marijuana Grower* [1] described Neil as a "rumpled old sage of a guy who has experience with what he does." Now Neil says that he is not exactly sure what Michael meant, but it sounded good at the time. Neil's best description of himself is:

A man who works with recovery… *provides the opportunity for those who choose, to see themselves differently* … a father, a grandfather, a friend to the friendless, and a person who has had to recover from his own recovery issues; an alcoholic and a newly married man.

---

1 Greystone Books – Douglas & McIntyre Toronto and Vancouver – page 137-145

Born in St. Thomas Ontario in 1947, he was raised in the classic dysfunctional home (they meant well, but...). Zooming ahead—he was married, widowed, re-married, divorced and recently remarried to Karen.

Over the years he did everything from working in the RCMP, both in the Criminal Investigation Branch and Security Services, to chanting at a yoga ashram on Paradise Island (*right beside Club Med . . . how handy*). He taught at and was Associate Director of Student Services at Twin Valley's School (TVS), Wardsville, Ontario:

An Alternative To The Penal System For Young Offenders. *TVS was very closely connected to Findhorne in Scotland. As Director of Student Services Neil worked very closely with the various levels of the Family Court System and Social Assistance Programs in Ontario, i.e. Metro Toronto Children's Aid, the Ontario Ministry of Health etc.*

Neil has authored, co-facilitated, and facilitated a number of different workshops and seminars on spiritual development and recovery:

- The Door --- A Workshop on Inner Self Discovery

- Zen and the Art of Lost and Found --- Workbook

- Zen and the Art of Walking Lightly --- Workbook

- Zen and the Art of Seeing Clearly --- Workbook

- Zen & the Art Of The 5 Principles of the Journey --- Workbook in editing.

- Experience Has Taught Us --- Searching for the Willingness to Change --- Steps 1->5

- A Step Four and Five Guide --- Workbook

- The Ghost and the Dustman, A Spy Novel

- Game On, A Spy Novel.

END NOTES

---

[i] Taken from **A Course In Miracles** ... Manuel for Teachers ... Page 9 ... On Trust ... Foundation for Inner Peace ...

[ii] Taken from **Experience Has Taught Us 175 Missing Pieces** Published Bright Star Press Author Neil Douglas-Tubb

[iii] Adapted from **How Can I Help** ... Ram Dass and Paul Gorman ... Publisher ... Knopf

[iv] From Quotes by **Arthur C Clarke** ... author ... futurist ... visionary

[v] Adapted From Quotes by Arthur C Clarke ...

[vi] From Quotes by **Arthur C Clarke ...** author ... futurist ... visionary

www.ingramcontent.com/pod-product-compliance
Lightning Source LLC
Chambersburg PA
CBHW051216250726
48655CB00006B/2432